Strokes of Color 2

An Adult Coloring Book for Stroke Survivors

Laura De La Cruz

For information, contact
Laura De La Cruz
75 County Road A074
Chaparral, NM 88081
professordelacruz@gmail.com

Dedication

The first "Strokes of Color" coloring book was designed at the request of my best friend Cynthia Gamez on behalf of her father. A stroke survivor, he needed a coloring book that allowed him to work on his motor skills and be successful when coloring or painting.

Unfortunately, we lost Mr. Brown before he was able to try out the coloring book. However, many stroke survivors have and they enjoyed expressing their artistic side.

This second book is dedicated to them and Mr. Brown. You are missed sir.

DANIEL HOWARD BROWN
SEPT 8, 1929 – OCT 5, 2016

How to use this coloring book

Please feel free to tear out the pages and put up for painting or coloring.

Each is simple but fun to fill.

Good luck!

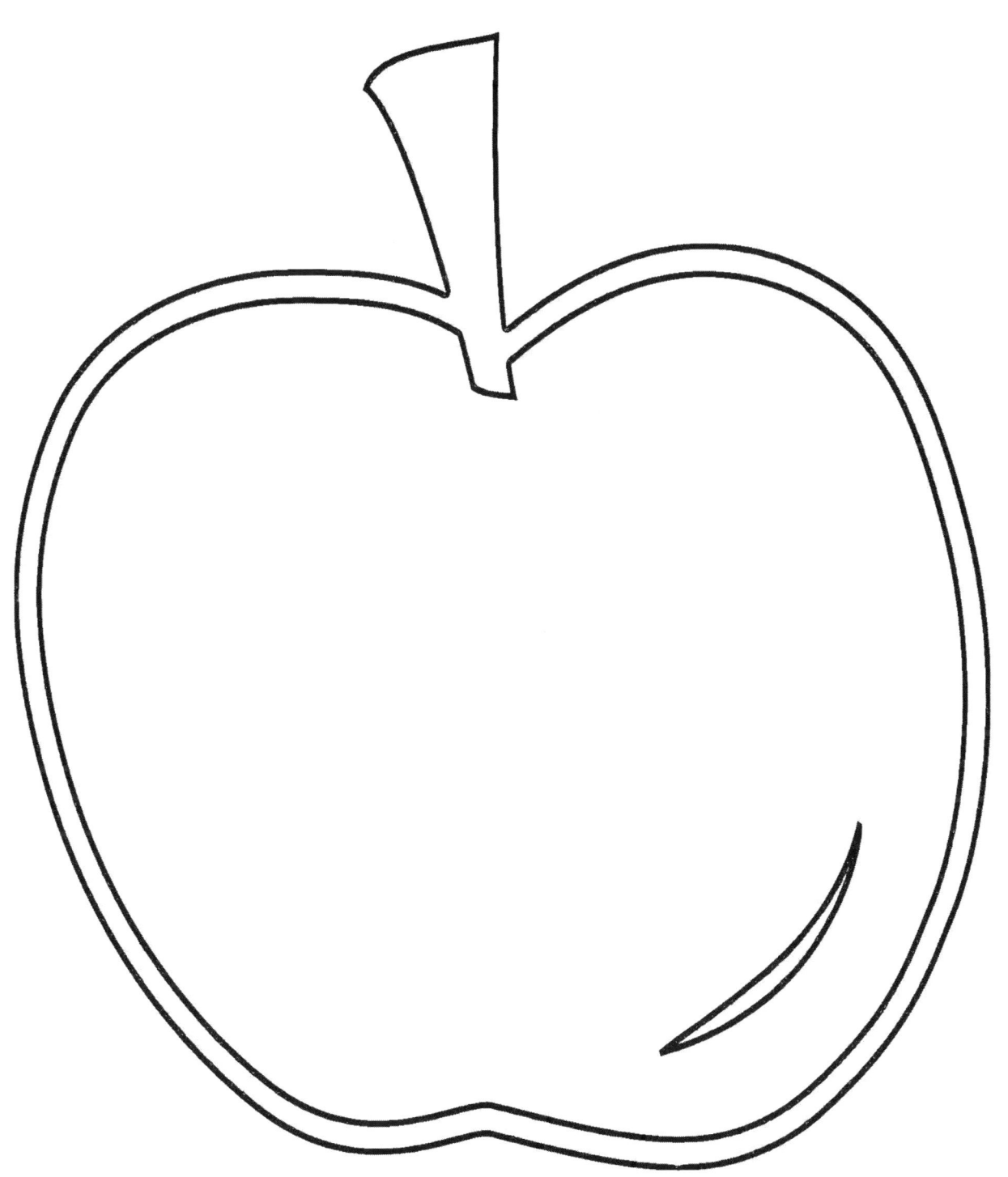

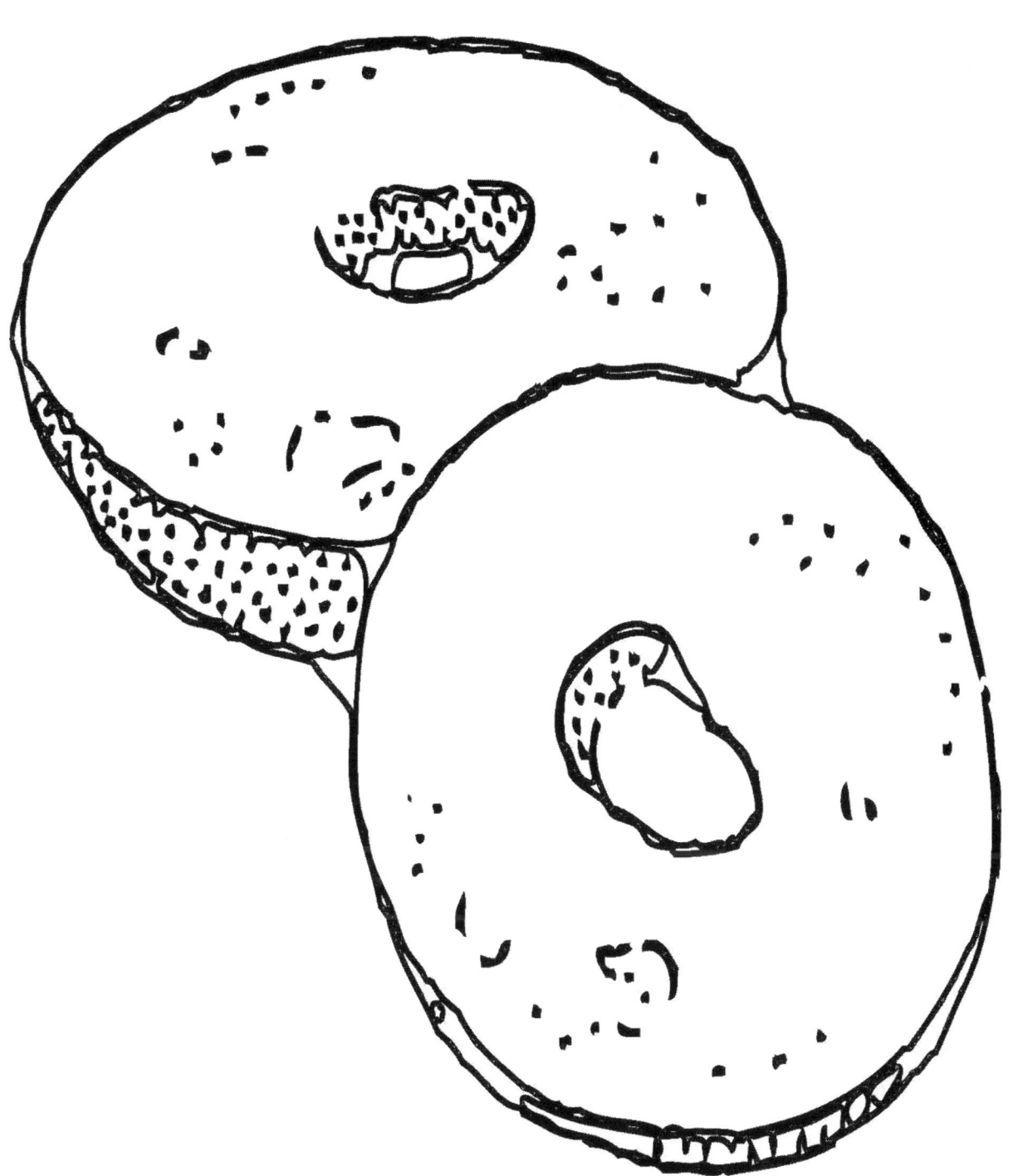

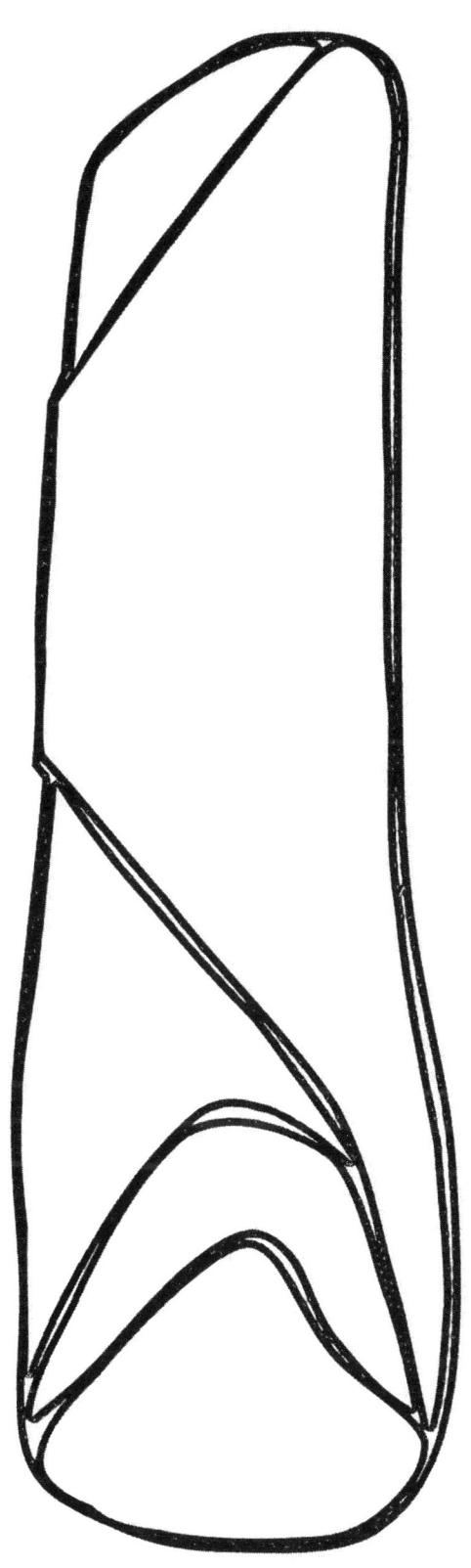

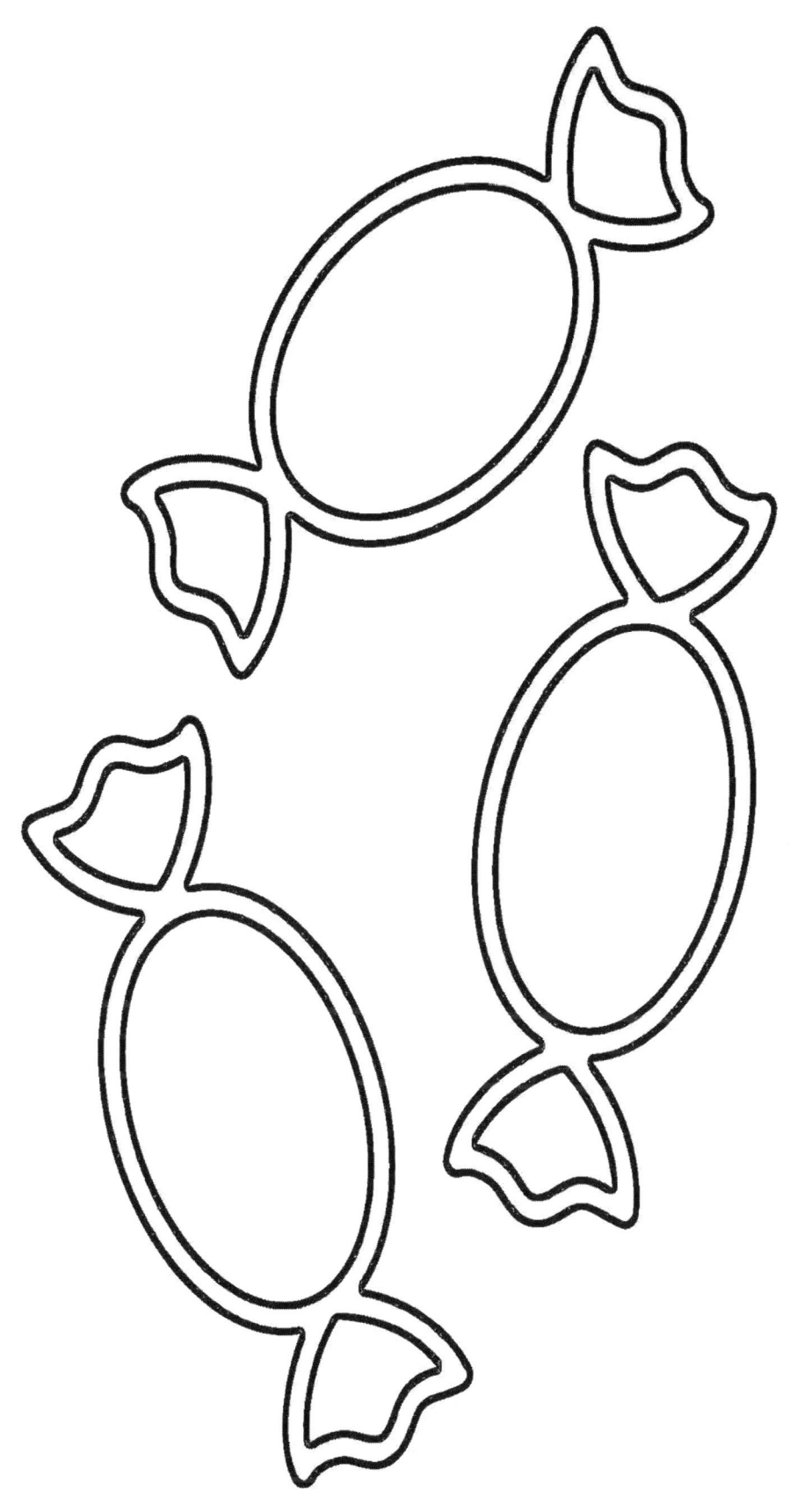

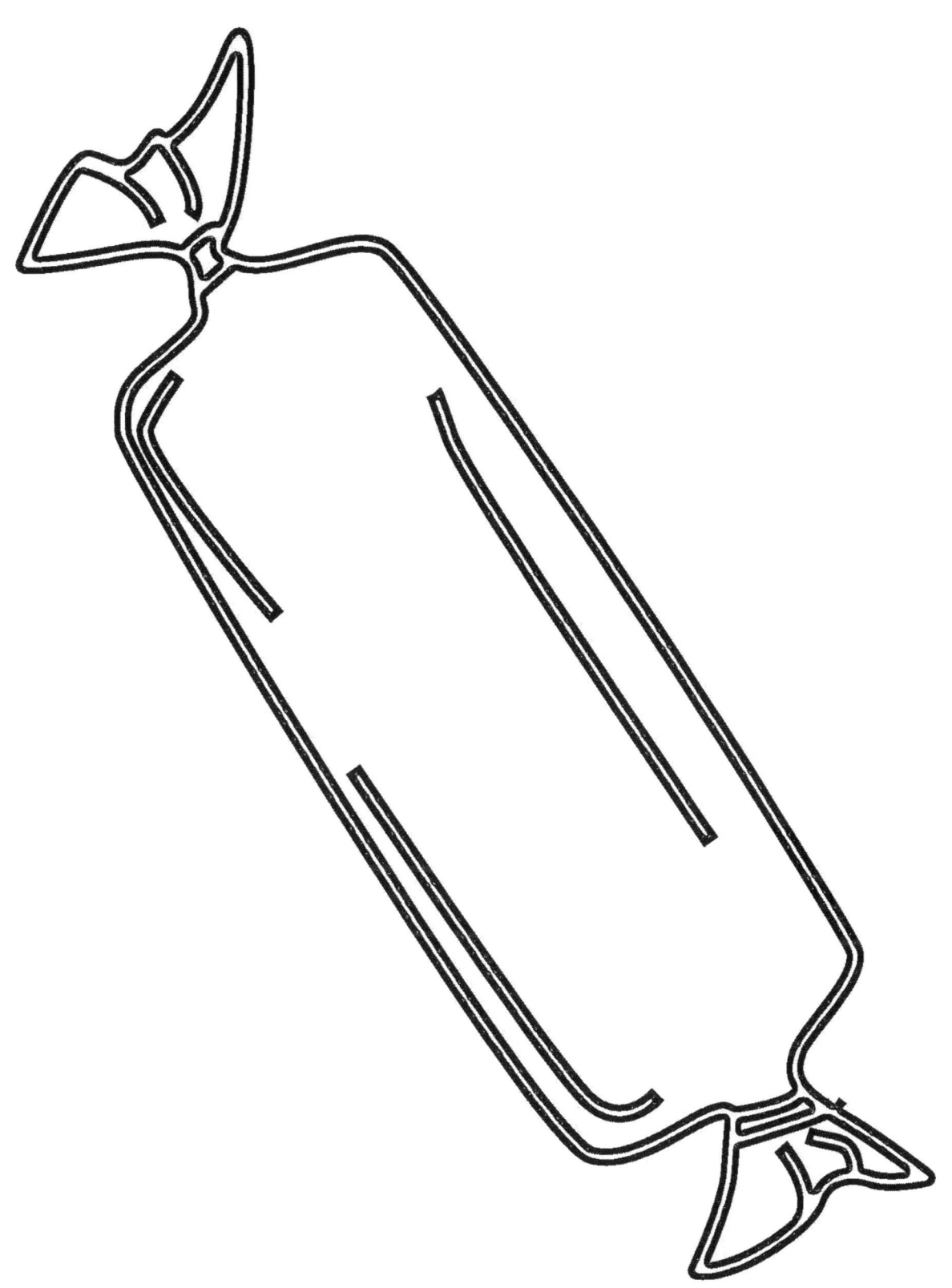

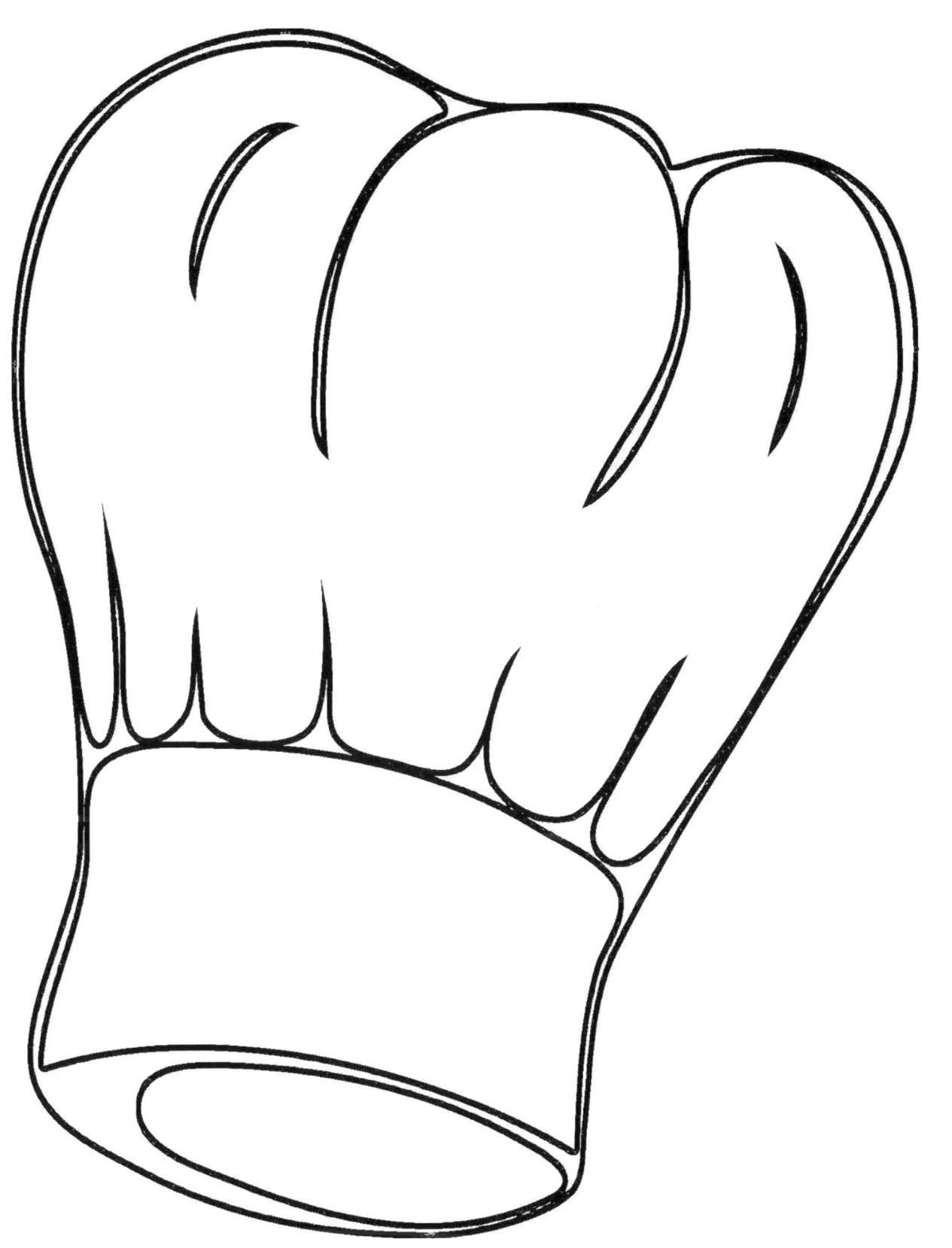

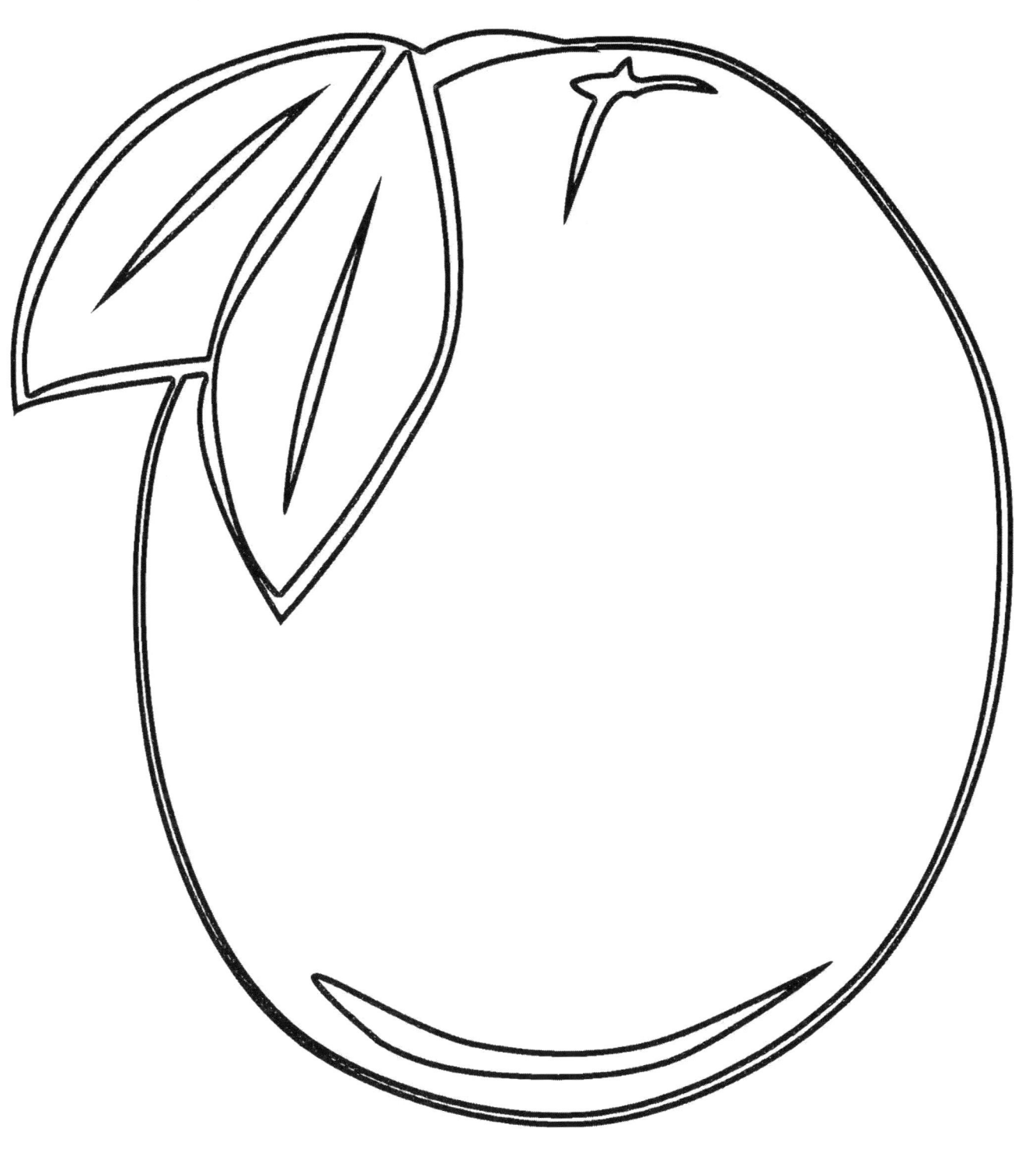

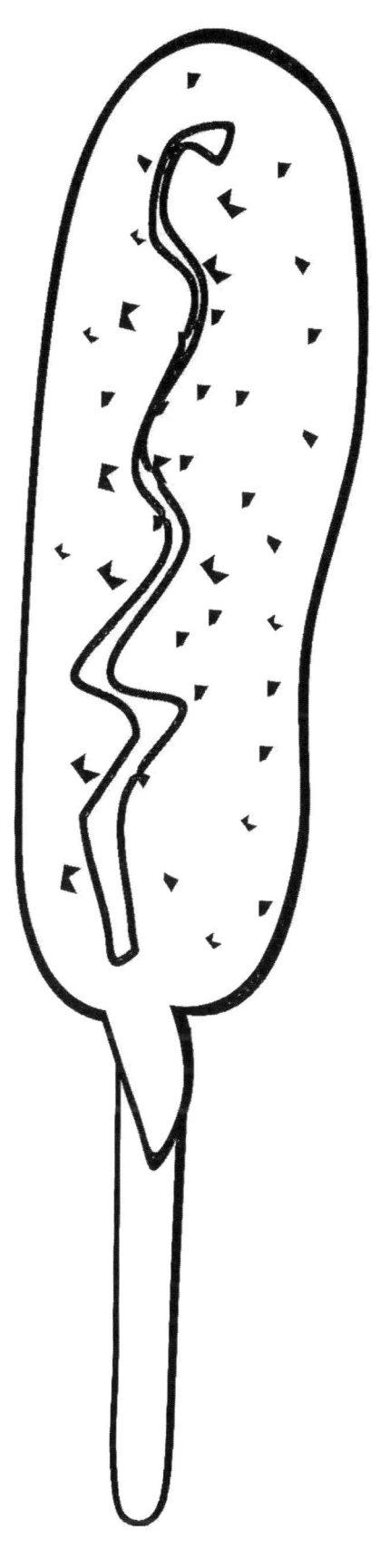

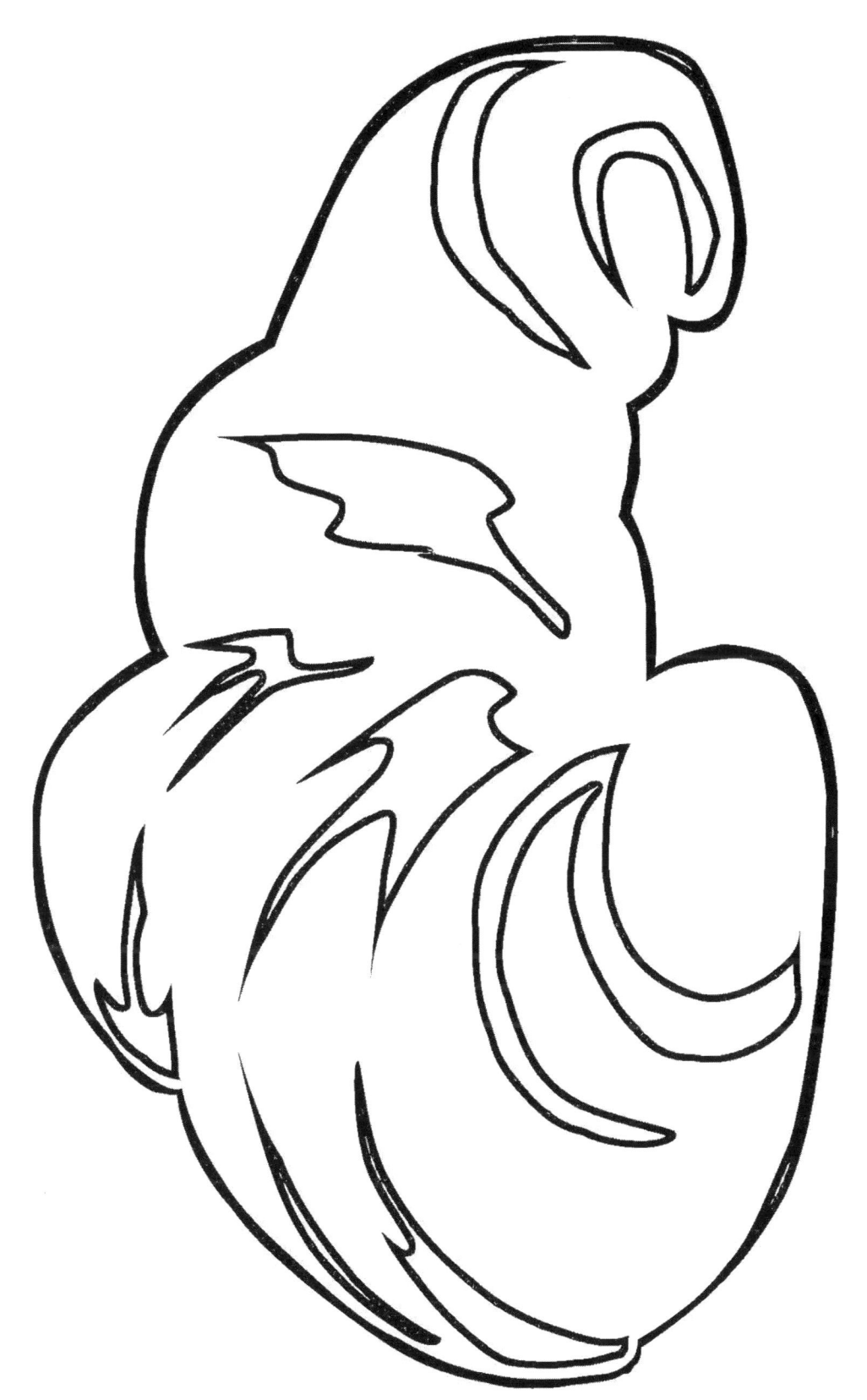

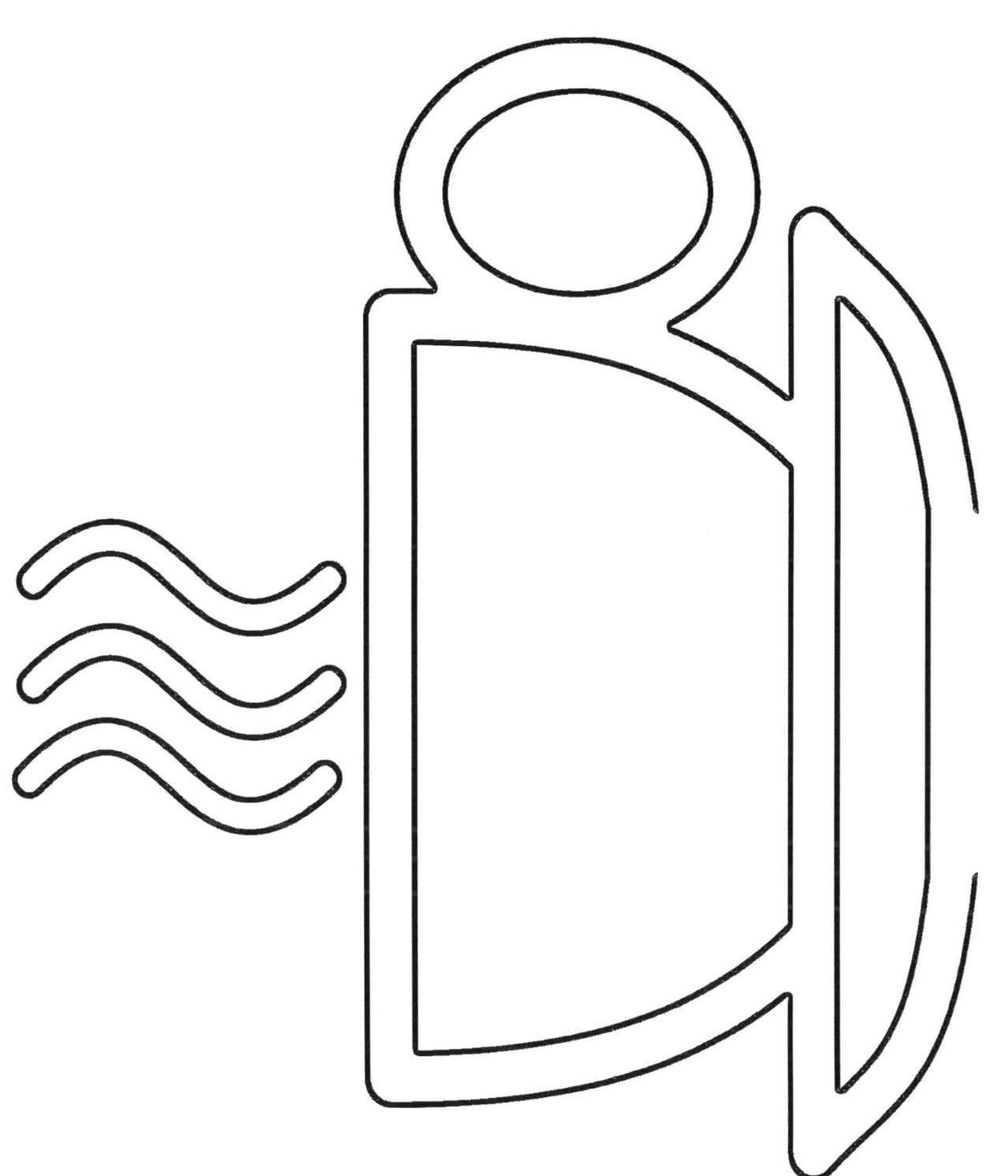

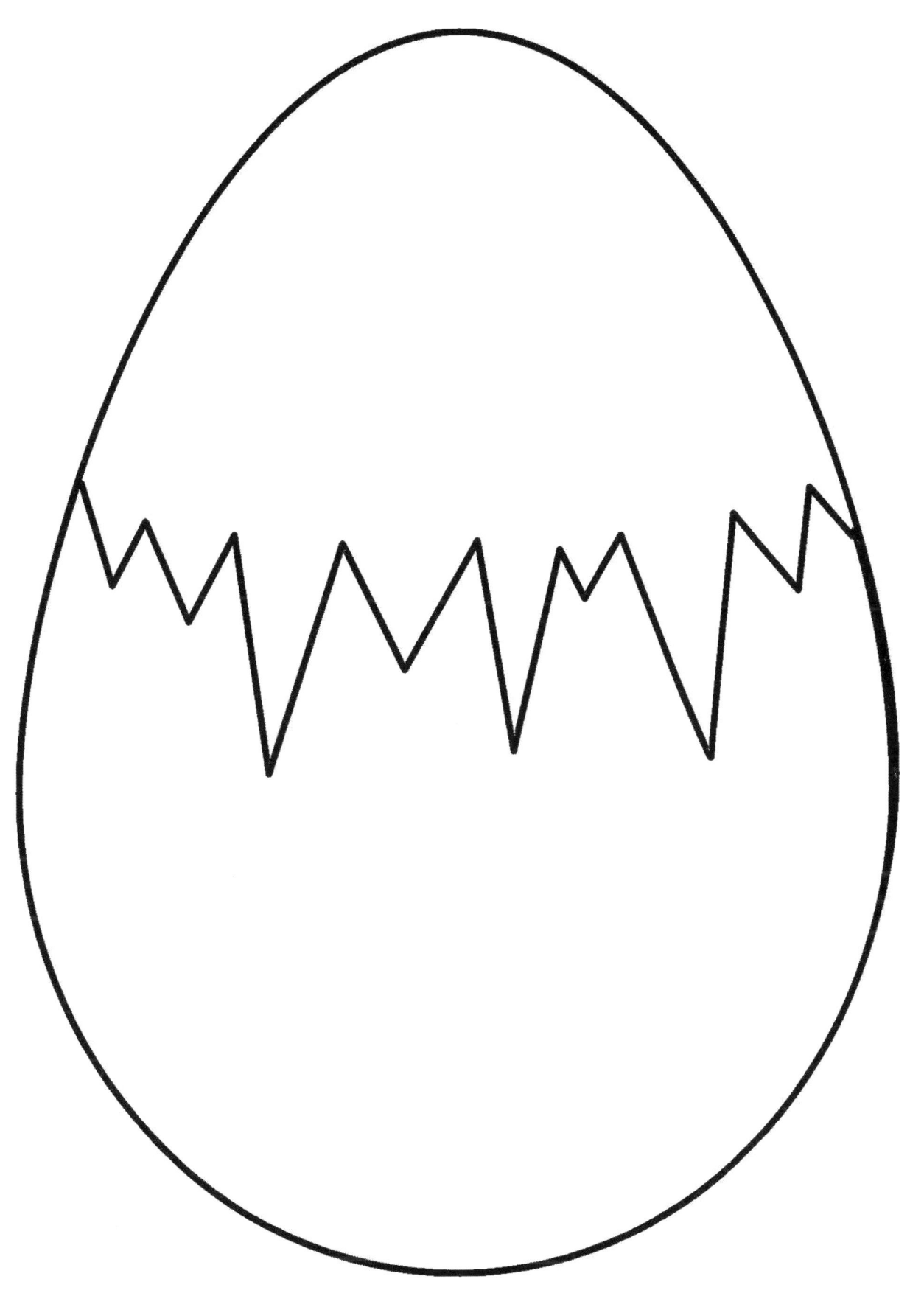

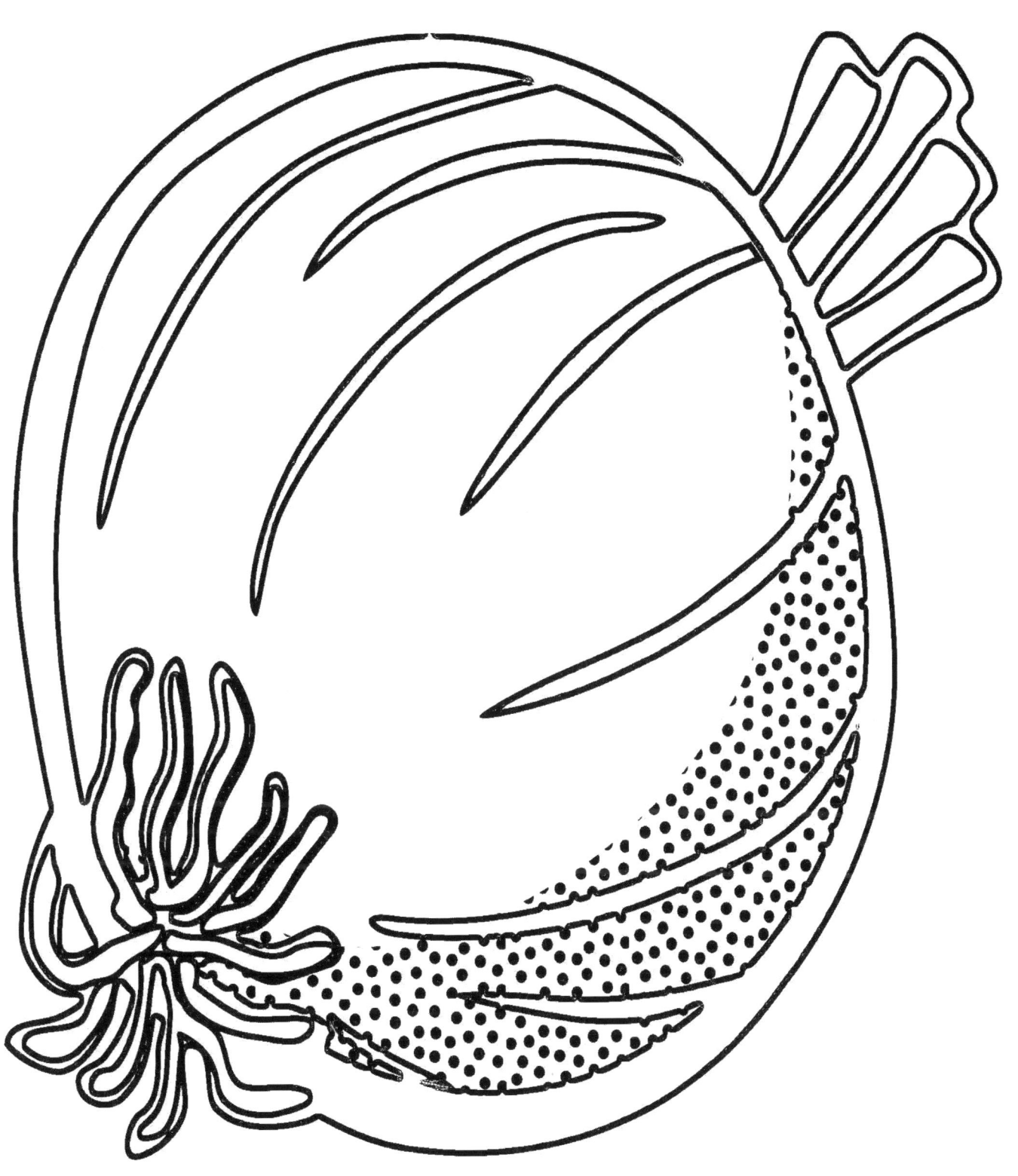

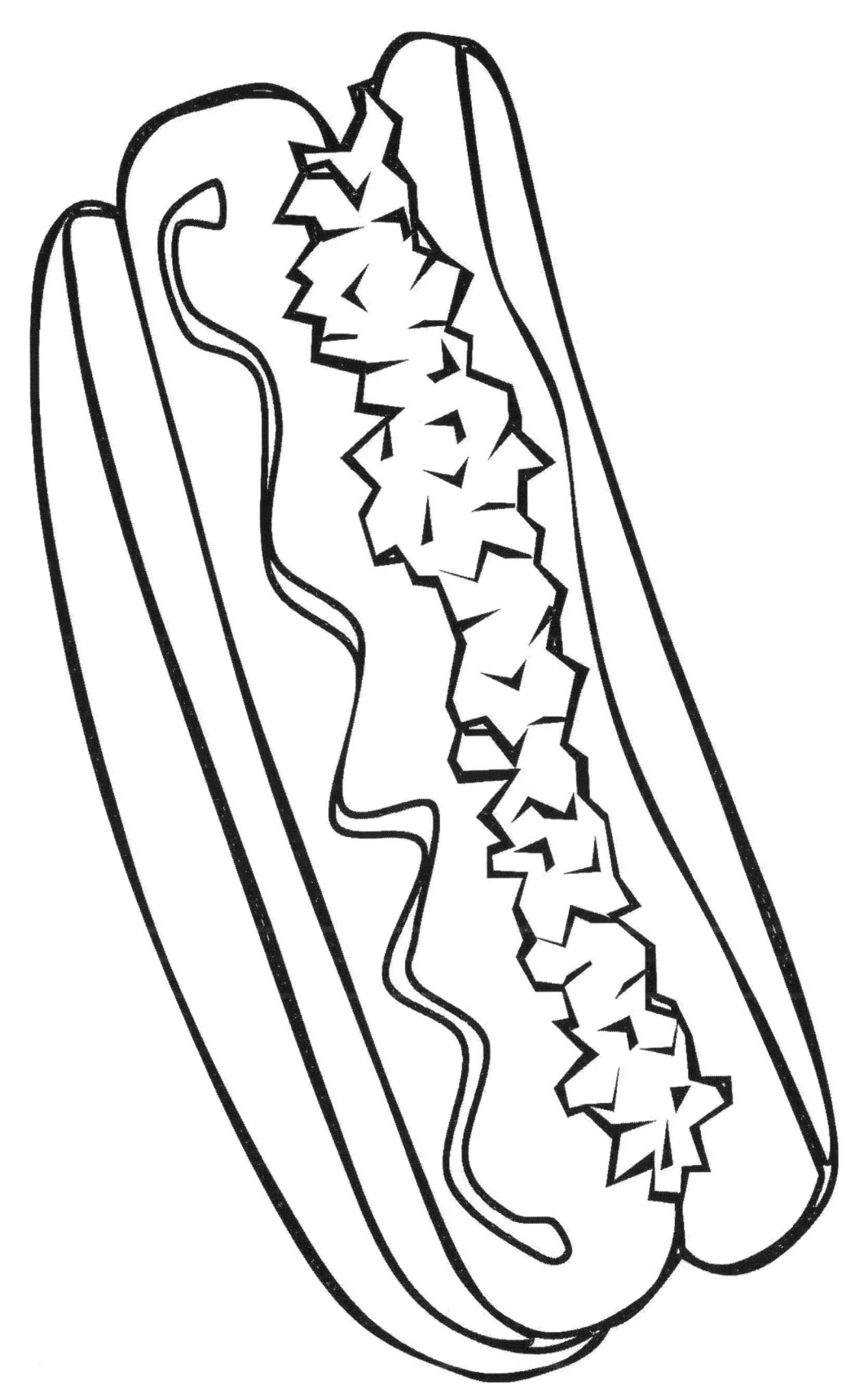

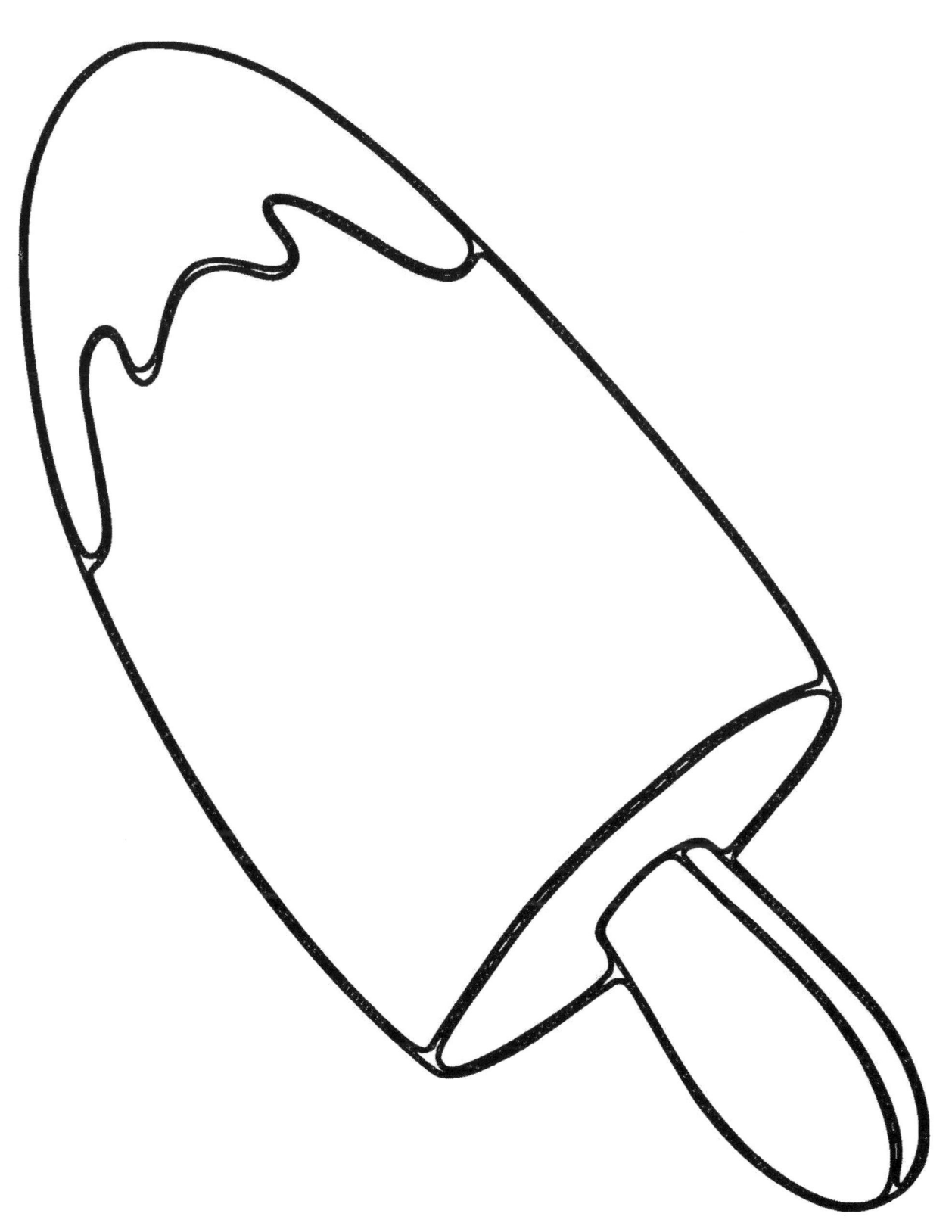

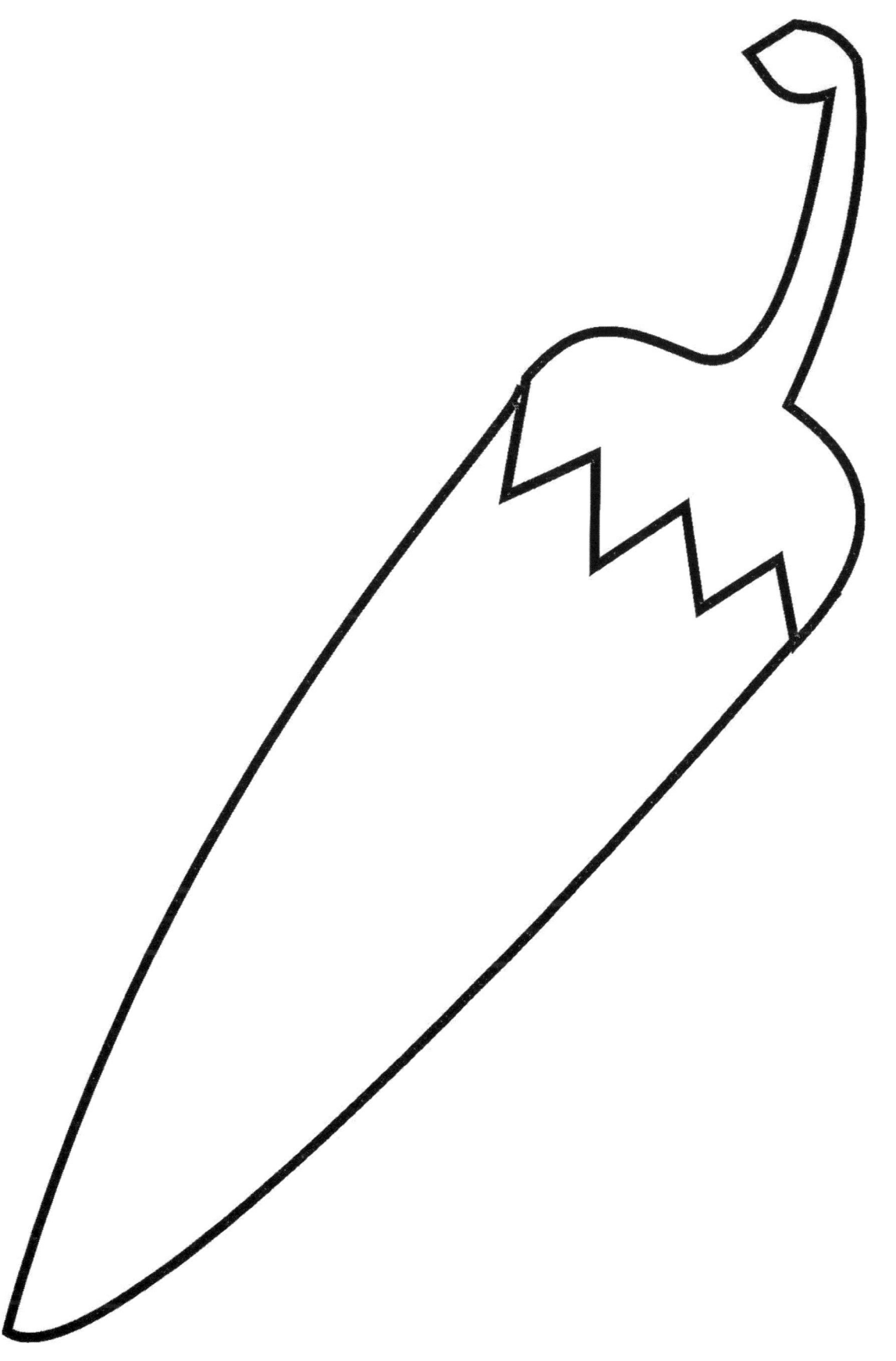

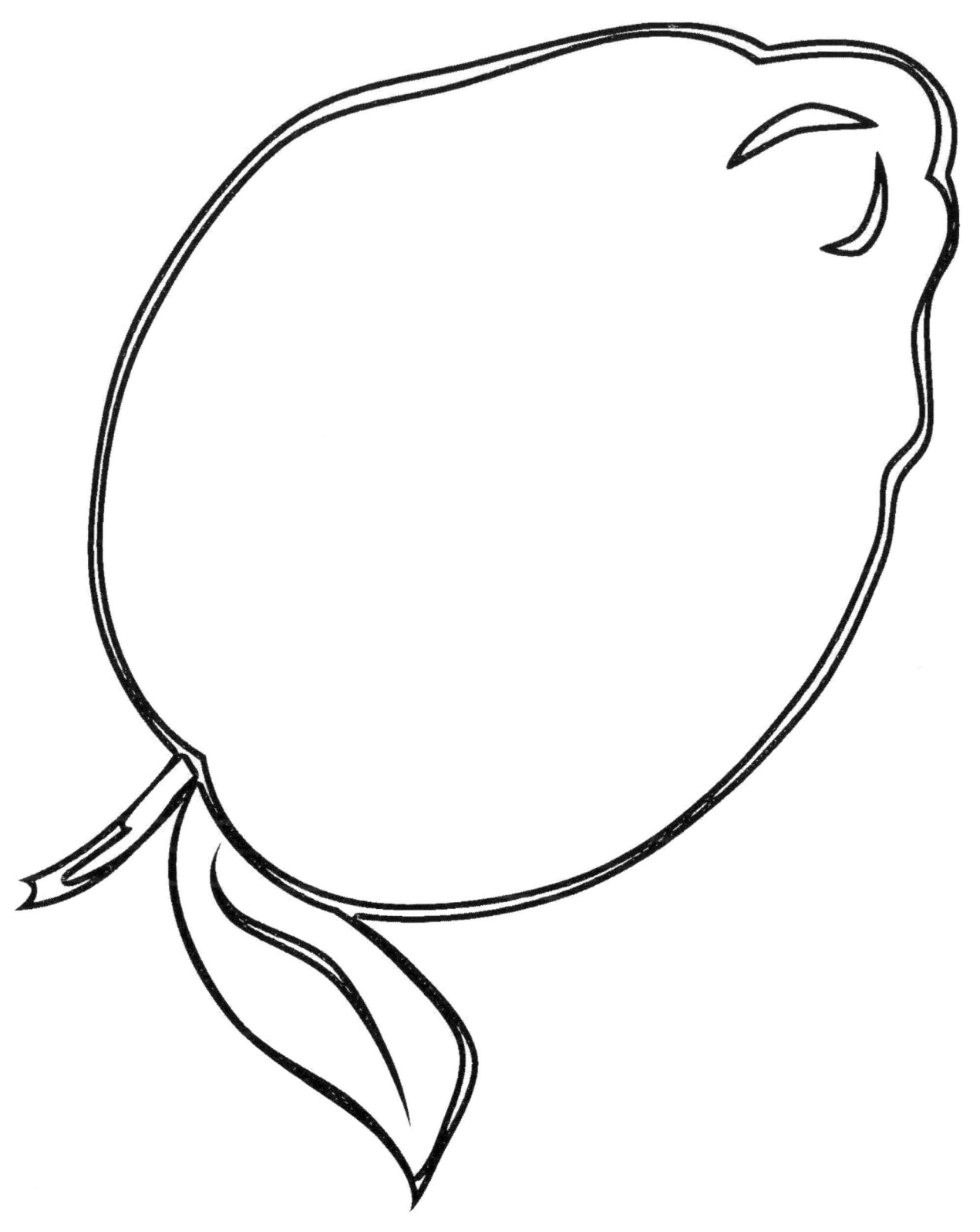

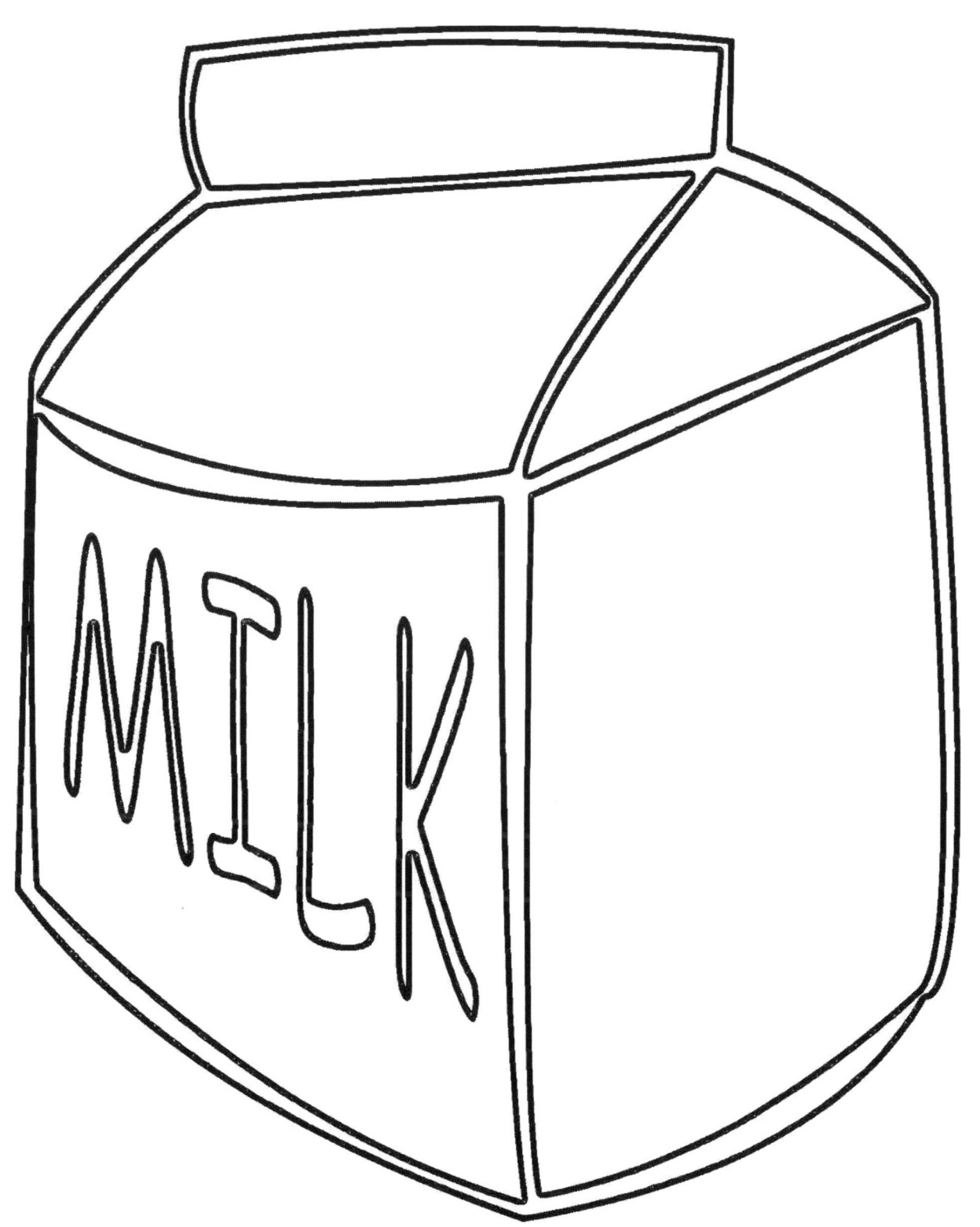

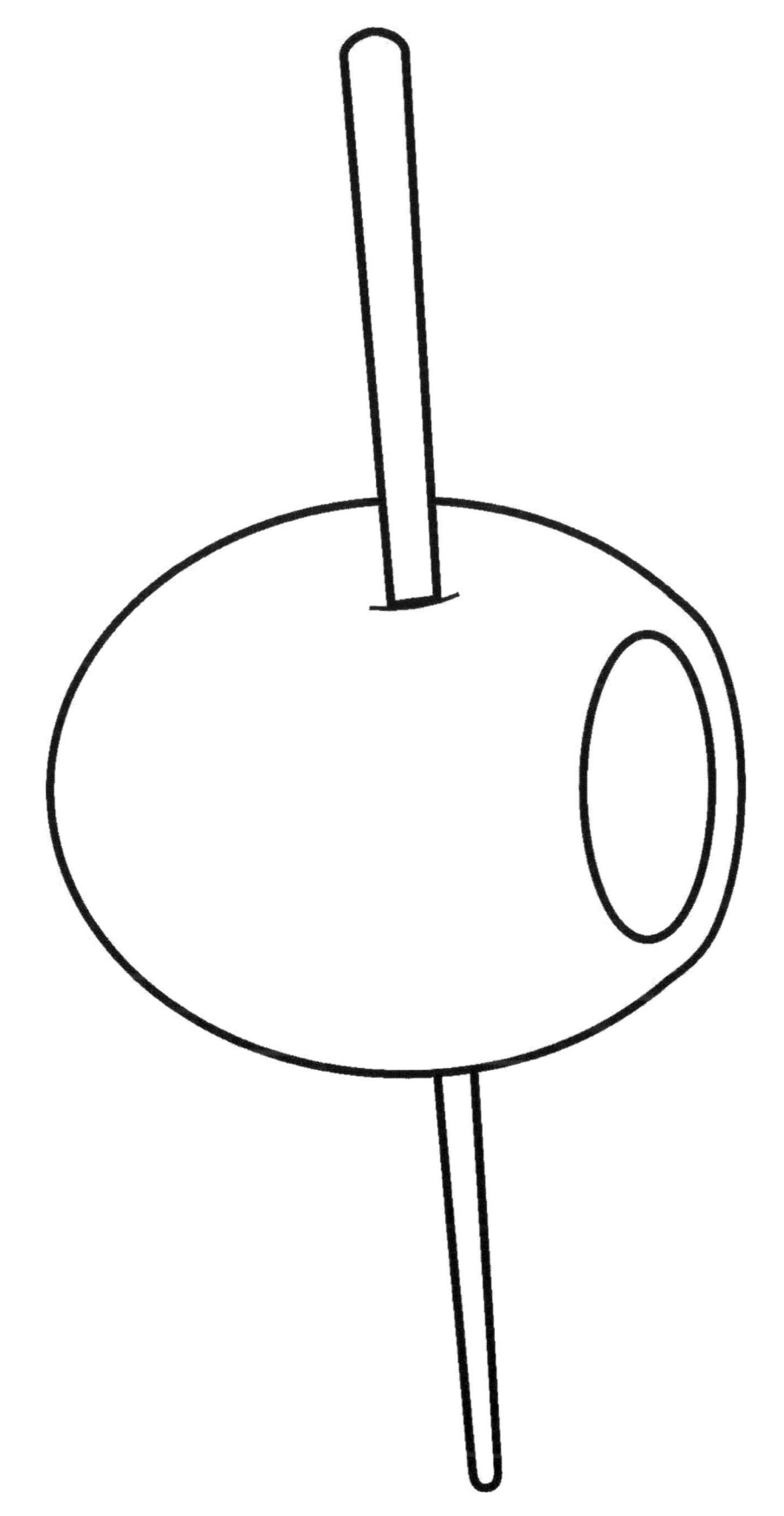

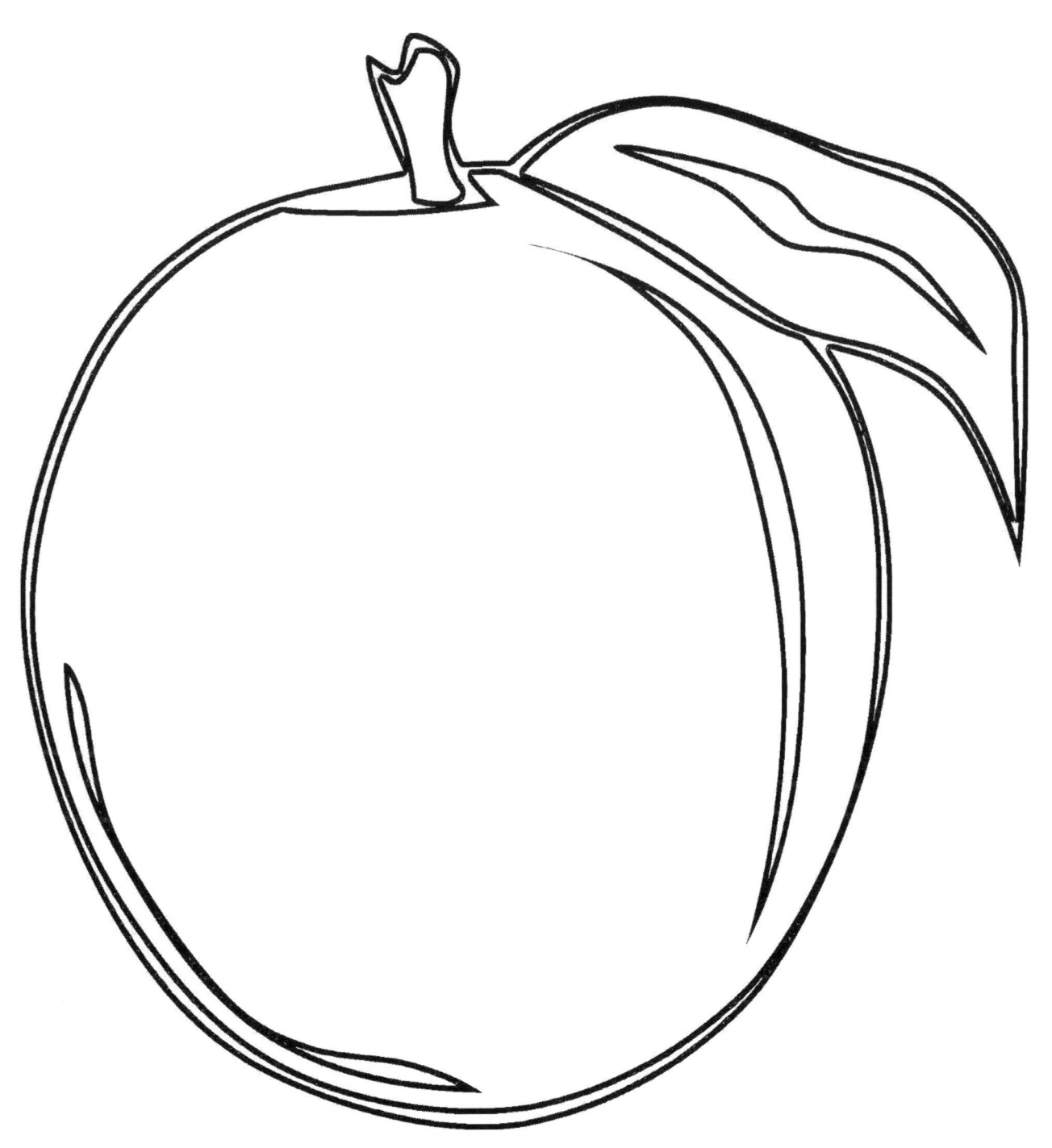

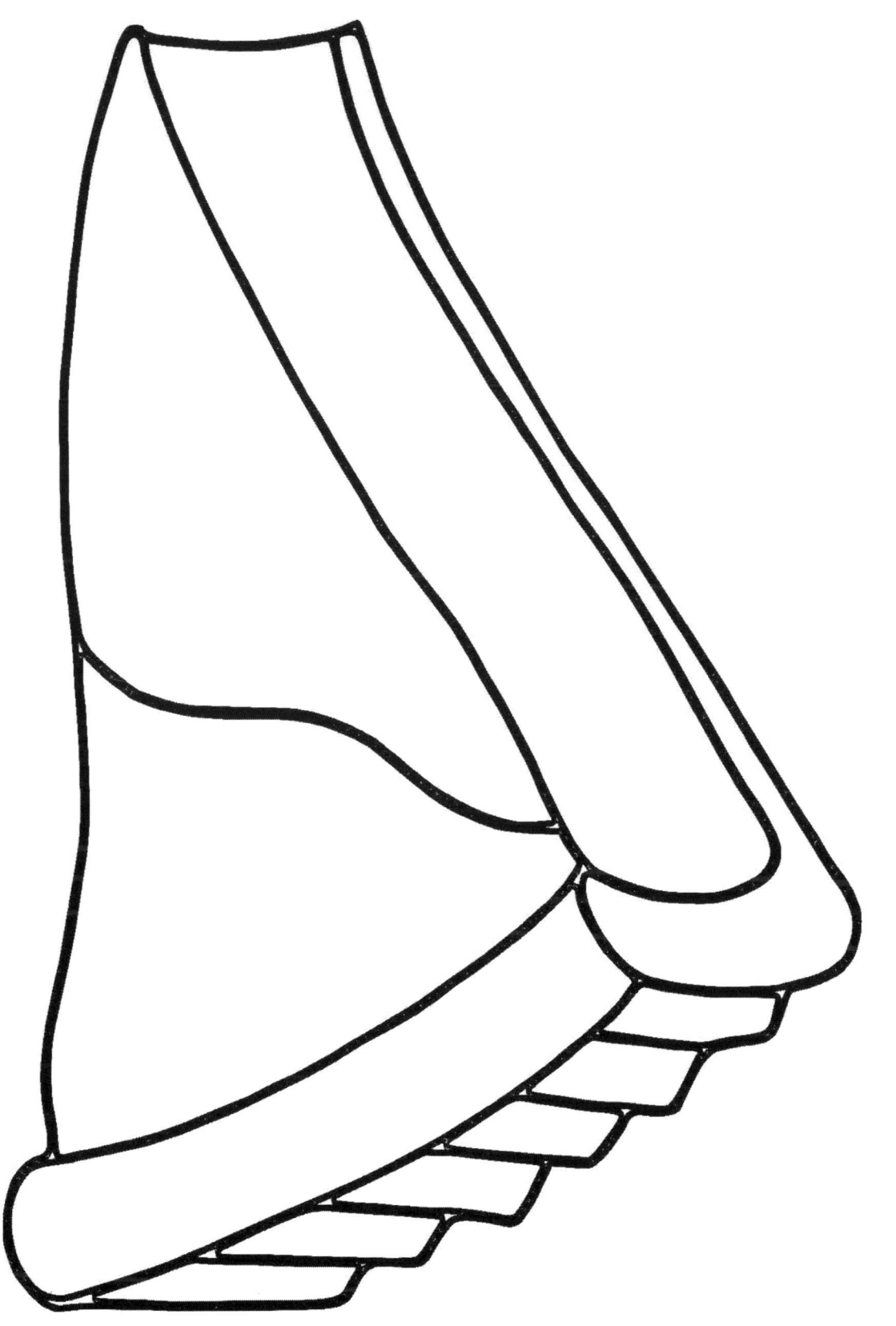

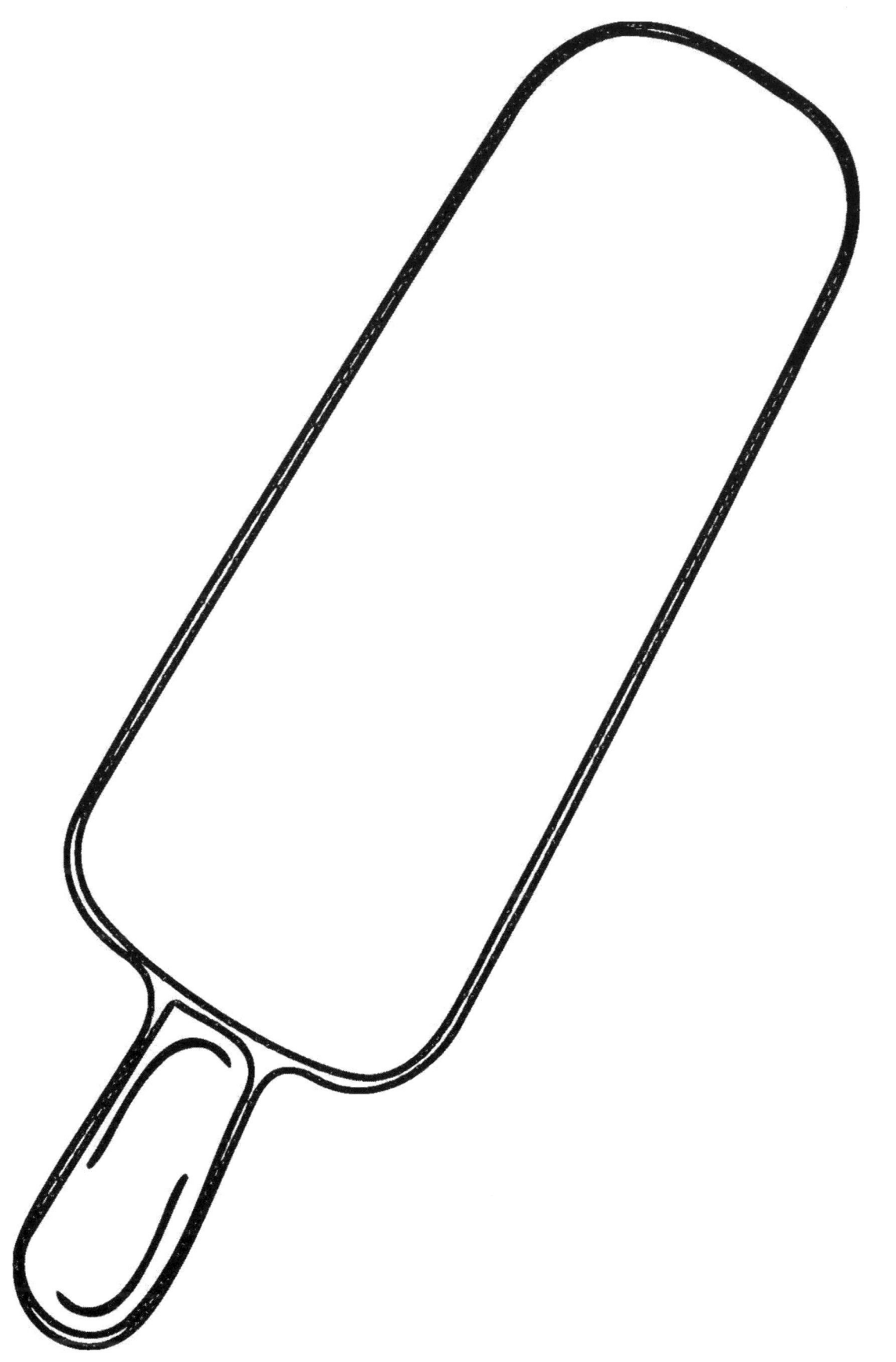

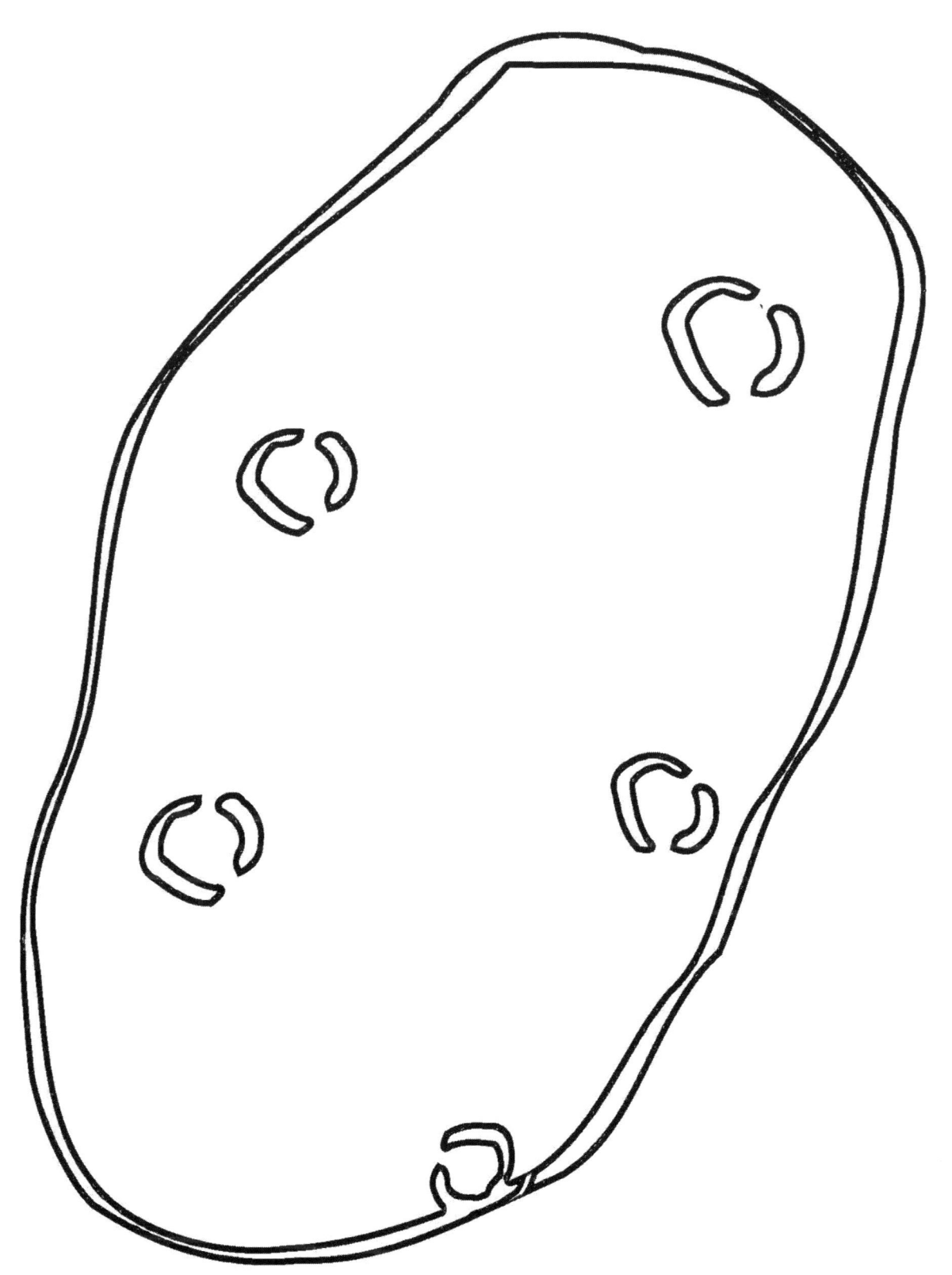

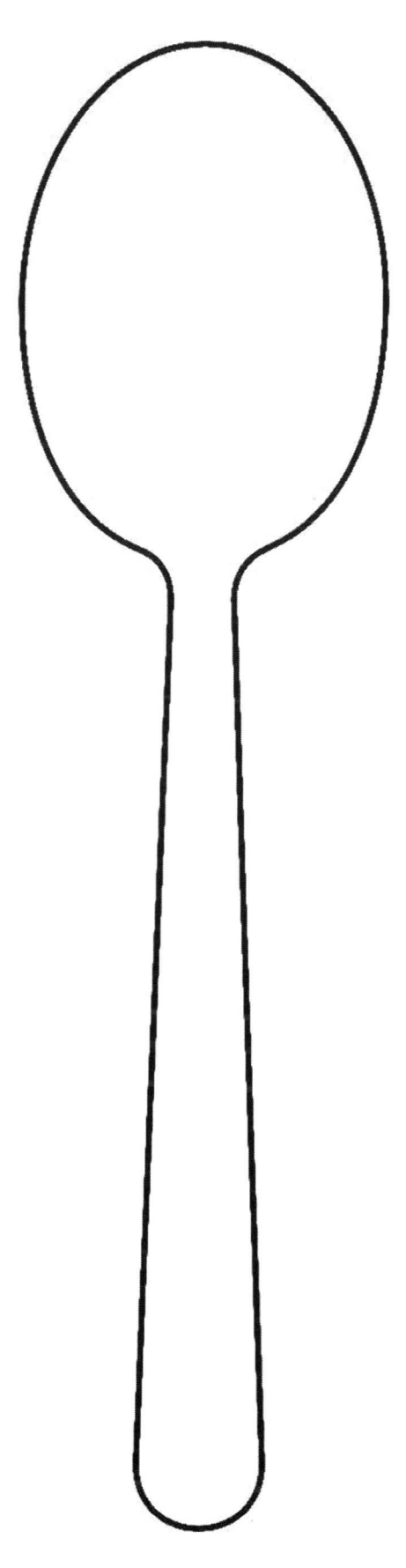

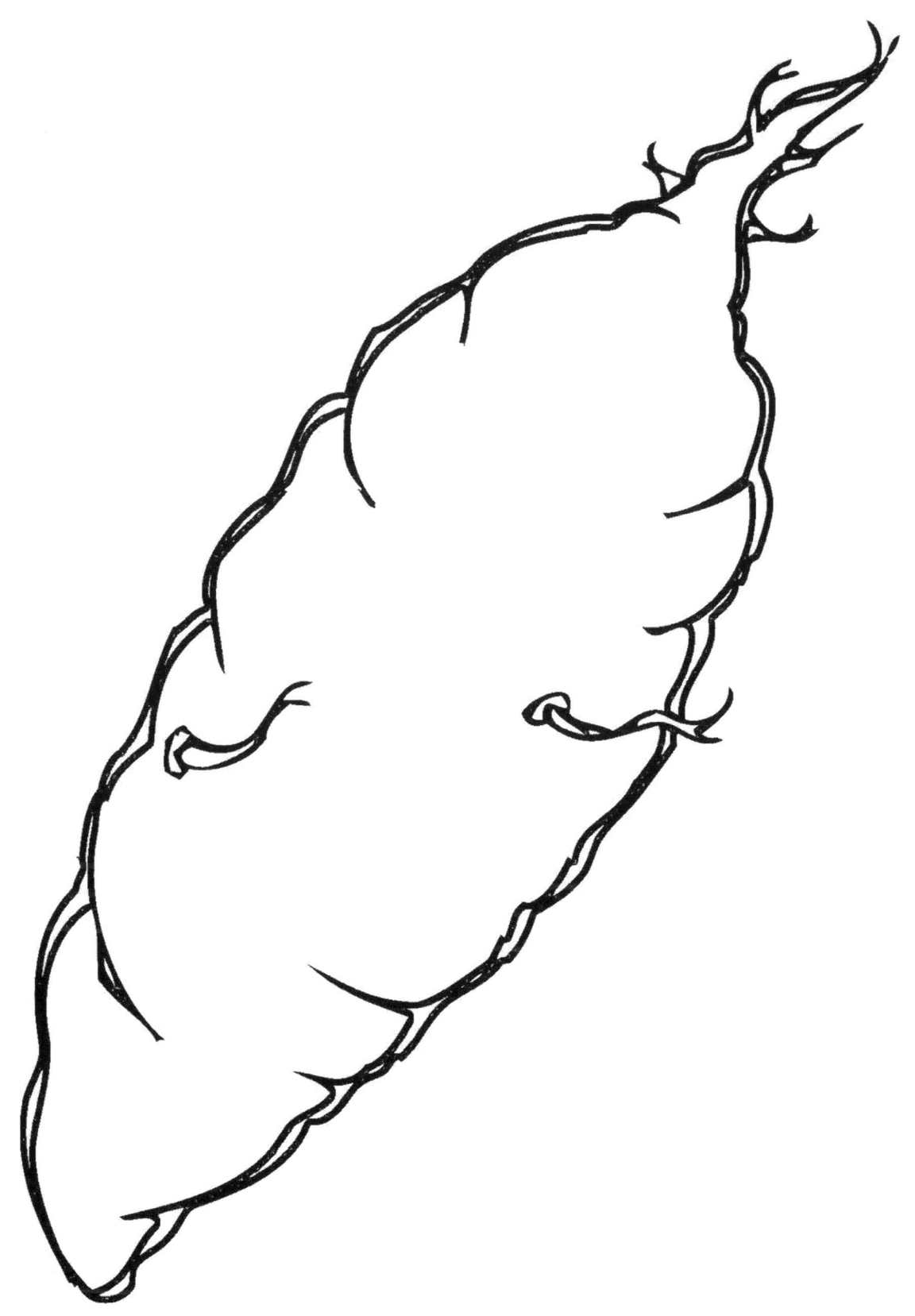

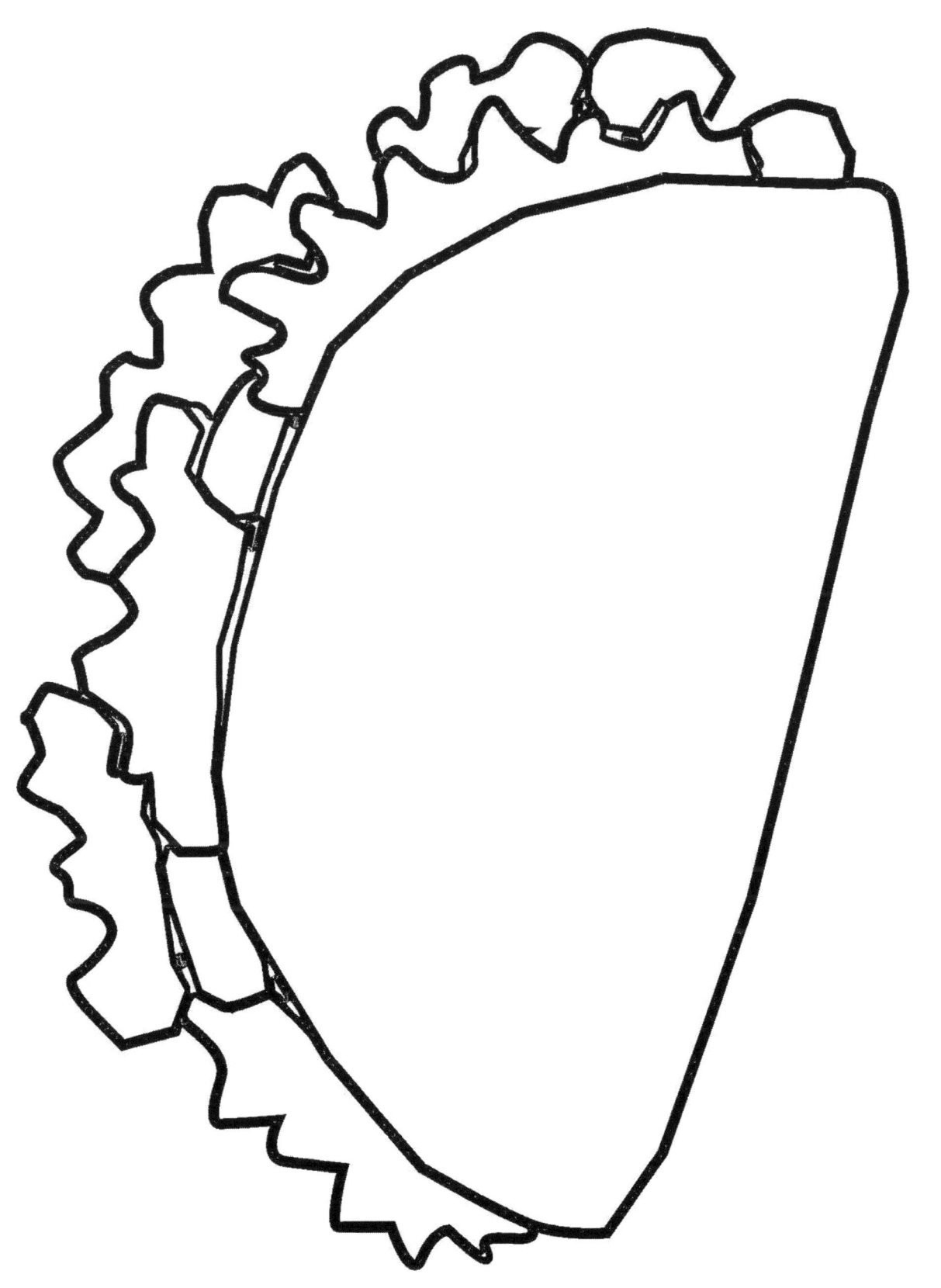

Thank you for purchasing this book. If you found it useful for your loved one, please leave a positive review on Amazon.

Our hope is that it helps. Your family is in our thoughts and prayers.

Laura & Cynthia

Printed in Great Britain
by Amazon